DOSAGE
CALCULATIONS
FOR NURSING STUDENTS

A COMPLETE STEP-BY-STEP GUIDE FOR QUICK DRUG DOSAGE CALCULATION. DOSING MATH TIPS & TRICKS FOR STUDENTS, NURSES, AND PARAMEDICS.

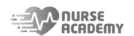

NURSE ACADEMY

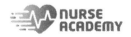

CONTENTS

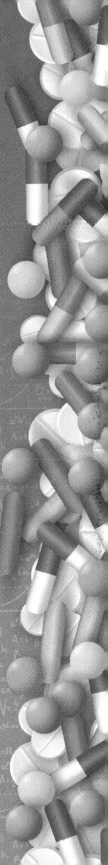

INTRODUCTION

Drug administration and prescription are some of the most important tasks performed by nurses, according to O'Shea, 1999. Errors in drug administration are a technical problem, despite the increased use of various tools and systems for the safe prescription and administration of drugs.

Appropriate administration of drugs requires an accurate calculation of doses. It is an important nursing skill and is vital for patient safety. According to international studies in literature, the rate of drug administration and dose calculation errors has been recorded as high.

The National Patient Safety Agency (NPSA) reported that 59.3% of drug administration errors occurred over the course of drug preparation. These errors comprise 28.7% of all reported drug errors. According to Wright, 2006, many drug administration errors arise from dose calculation errors, as a result of the arithmetic attitude towards the calculation of drugs by nurses.

These calculation errors may arise either from the inability to perform simple arithmetic operations, like the four arithmetic operations and mathematics with

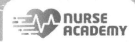

fractional numbers and decimal numbers, or from neglect of the required data needed for generating correct equations.

Based on international reports of adverse drug events, incorrect doses account for up to one-third of these events. Most health professionals find drug calculations difficult.

Studies have also indicated that nursing students have poor medication dose calculation and arithmetic skills. In their study of 66 nursing students in the USA, Blais and Bath (1992) determined that 89% of nursing students failed drug calculation tests and had difficulties calculating the correct dose.

Jukes and Gilchrist (2006) assessed sophomore nursing students and showed similar results.

Dilles et al. (2011) indicated limited calculation skills knowledge in pharmacology by nursing students. McMullan et al. (2010) emphasized that 92% of 229 nursing students in England failed a drug calculation test. The research suggested that efforts to improve essential numerical and drug calculation skills should be included in the university curriculum.

Niemi et al. (2001) stated that the students had difficulties learning mathematical and drug calculation skills from a study conducted with the aim of determining the basic mathematical sufficiency and drug dose calculation skills of 204 nursing students who had graduated in Finland, Grendel. From this study, students

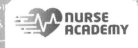

were found to have insufficient mathematical skills, while one-fifth of them failed a drug calculation test.

Further studies have evaluated the students' basic mathematical skills and determined that 158 second-year nursing students had insufficient skills, particularly in the division, formula use, and multiplication of fractional numbers.

During the same study, the students were subjected to a test of 10 items related to commonly used clinical calculations. Only 55% of the students were able to answer all of the questions correctly.

Brown (2002) found similar results when a basic mathematical test was administered to 868 nursing students in the USA.

Various Departments of Health have established that drug calculation skills are important for patients and have suggested that more research should be performed on drug dose calculation errors in clinical practice.

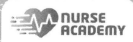

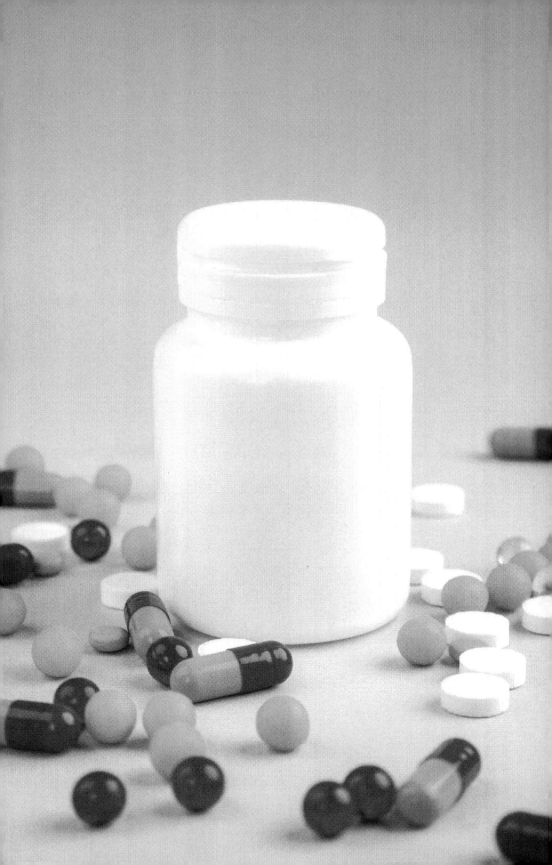

WHAT ARE DRUGS?

Drugs are chemicals that interact with proteins to affect a physio-logical function. Scholars and scientists have come up with other definitions to explain drugs as a substance used in the diagnosis, treatment, and/or prevention of diseases or a component of a medication (Houghton Mifflin, 2004).

When these substances are absorbed into the body, they bind with certain pro-teins, causing a slight change in the functioning of the cell.

COMPONENTS OF DRUGS

A drug functions through the body when the active ingredient is released. The amount of chemical needed to cause an effect in most drugs is very small, often up to 5 mg.

Most drugs that we take also have inactive_ingredients that act as fillers of the drugs. These ingredients have no effect on the functioning of cells, and when administered orally, bind the drug and lubricate it to make it easy to swallow.

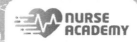
NURSE ACADEMY

Hence, these ingredients act as fillers, binders, and lubricants of the drug while the active ingredients, whose chemicals are in small amounts, react with the body to produce the results.

HOW DRUGS WORK

Human bodies largely rely on proteins. These proteins exist in several forms with different functions. Each protein has a specific function and is quite specific to the cell type that it acts on.

There is a type of protein called receptors. These proteins are embedded on the surfaces of the cells which are also for different types of cells. This receptor joins other proteins and chemicals outside the cell which in turn creates a change in how the cell functions.

Proteins are drug targets. For a drug to be effective it needs to be joined to a protein. To unlock its effectiveness, the proteins act as the lock and the drugs as the key such that, when the two bind, the proteins are unlocked to produce a change in response.

THE EFFECTS OF DRUGS ON THE BODY

Drugs produce therapeutic effects once they are joined with the proteins in the body. The main stages that take place when the drugs enter the body include

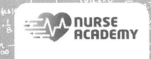

absorption, distribution, metabolism, and excretion.

The drug is absorbed into the blood to enter the cells; this is followed by the distribution of the drug in the body. The drug then breaks down, a process called metabolism, and lastly excretion of the drug from the body takes place.

ASSESSING THE RISKS AND BENEFITS OF DRUGS

Some medications have side effects on the functioning of the body in addition to what they are intended to treat. At this stage, a patient and a doctor or physician have to work together to determine the risks and benefits of the administered medication.

To determine the risks, patients must tell their doctors which drugs or medications they are on (including herbal supplements), any allergies they have, and any previous effects they have experienced from the medication.

It is important that patients keep track of the medications they are taking, their function, and the risks that come with them. They should ask their doctors if there are any supplements to a specific drug if what they have been given before has had adverse side effects. Nurses and doctors should discourage patients from stopping a medication without the advice and direction of a physician.

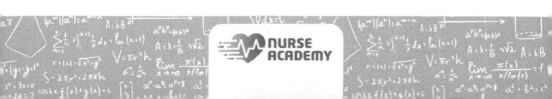

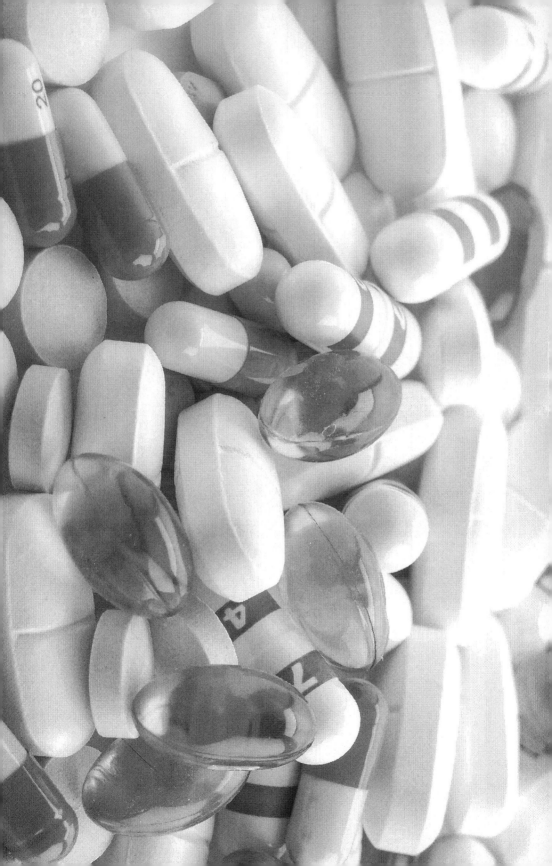

CLASSIFICATION OF DRUGS

This chapter will discuss the major classifications of drugs.

PHARMACOLOGIC

These are drugs with similar characteristics and containing similar chemical make-up and describe a drug's properties in a specific way and are necessary when determining treatment. In addition, this classification often has the same suffix. Examples in this category include Penicillin and Beta Blockers

Pharmacological Class	Identifying Suffix
Benzodiazepines	"-epam" example Diazepam
Monoclonal Antibodies	"-map" example Rituximab
5-HT$_3$ Antagonists	"-setron" example Ondansetron

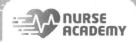

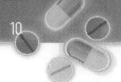

THERAPEUTIC

These are drugs that are used for similar effects and may not have a similar chemical makeup. These are based on therapeutic intent. Examples in this category include Antihypertensive and Antibiotics.

ALLOPATHIC

Allopathy is the principle of fighting or curing disease through administering a substance that produces the opposite effect of the disease when administered to a healthy person. This classification has been broken further to:

NON-PRESCRIPTION DRUGS

These are drugs that can be purchased from a pharmacy without the prescription of a doctor. They are also called over-the-counter drugs

ANTI-HEMORRHOID DRUGS

These are medicines that when administered, help to reduce the swelling and relieve the distress of hemorrhoids. They can be found as creams, ointments, and suppositories. These types of drugs can also be purchased without the doctor's prescription.

TOPICAL ANTIBIOTICS

These are medicines that can be applied to skin to fight or kill bacteria and help

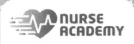

prevent infections caused by bacteria that get into minor cuts, burns, and scrapes. For quicker healing, wounds are treated with antibiotics, and if untreated, bacteria will multiply and cause pain, redness, swelling, itching, and oozing.

COUGH SUPPRESSANTS

These are medicines that help in preventing and stopping flu and coughs. They act in the center of the brain that controls the cough reflex and are meant to be used only to relieve dry, hacking coughs brought about by colds and flu. However, these drugs are not recommended in treating coughs that come with mucus or are associated with smoking, asthma, emphysema, or other lung conditions.

ANTI-ACNE DRUGS

These are medicines that clear up body spots and rushes like pimples, blackheads, whiteheads, and other forms of acne. There are several categories under this classification that depend on what is being fought. For example, lotions and soaps containing benzoyl peroxide which are used to treat mild to moderately severe acne.

NON-STEROIDAL ANTI-INFLAMMATORY DRUGS (NSAIDS)

These medicines act as pain relievers for swellings, stiffness, and inflammations. They are often prescribed for painful conditions including arthritis, tendinitis, sprains, strains, and gout among other injuries. Despite relieving pain, these drugs do not cure diseases or injuries causing the diseases.

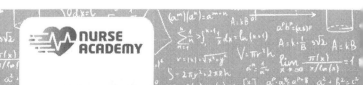

ANTISEPTICS

These are medicines that are applied to stop the growth of germs and help prevent infections in minor injuries like cuts and scrapes. They are normally applied to the skin to prevent bacteria from getting into wounds and causing infections. They only function by weakening bacteria and slowing their growth, not killing them.

ANALGESICS

These are pain relievers, prescribed to relieve pain of all types including headaches, backaches, joint pain, and those that result from surgery or injury. The most common drugs in this category include aspirin, sodium salicylate, choline salicylate, and magnesium salicylate.

Acetaminophen provides pain relief but does not reduce inflammation.

VASODILATORS

These are medicines that are applied and act directly on muscles in blood vessel walls to make blood vessels dilate. They are often used to treat hypertension by widening the arteries to allow blood to flow through easily.

EXPECTORANTS

These are drugs that loosen mucus and phlegm from the respiratory tract. Most cough medicines, including Anti-Tuss, Gaia, and Dristan Cold have guaifenesin as

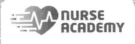

an ingredient. Drugs containing guaifenesin are only available upon a physician's prescription.

ANTIHISTAMINES

These are medicines that block compounds released in allergic inflammatory reactions at the H1 receptor sites and are responsible for immediate hypersensitivity reactions like sneezing and itching. The drugs reduce capillary fragility, which produces erythema or redness, associated with allergic reactions by inhibiting the activity of histamine. These drugs can also reduce histamine-induced secretions, including excessive tears and salivation.

ANTACIDS

These are drugs that neutralize stomach acid and are often used to relieve acid indigestion, upset stomach, sour stomach, and heartburn. Some contain the ingredient simethicone which relieves gas. They are taken by mouth and neutralize excess stomach acid. Antacids contain aluminum hydroxide and calcium bicarbonate in various combinations.

SALICYLATES

These are drugs that act as a pain reliever and also reduce fever. An example is aspirin which is used to relieve many kinds of minor aches and falls under sodium salicylate, choline salicylate, and magnesium salicylate.

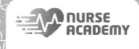

ANTI-FUNGAL

These are medicines that treat fungal infections. Most fungi are not very harmful. A few cause irritating infections while others cause much more severe infections. However, cancer and AIDS patients with compromised immune systems are more susceptible to fungal infections.

ANTIGAS AGENTS

These are medicines that relieve the uncomfortable symptoms of too much gas in the stomach and help relieve these symptoms by preventing the formation of pockets and breaking up gas that is already trapped in the stomach. These agents come as either capsules, liquids, or tablets and do not require a physician's prescription.

SMOKING CESSATION

These drugs are taken by tobacco and cigarette smokers to help them stop their consumption. These people often have a difficult time quitting smoking. The cessation products under this category contain nicotine, which is administered in small, steady doses spread out over several hours.

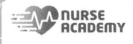

METROLOGY

DEFINING METROLOGY

Metrology is the science of measurements. In medicine and especially in critical care, frequent confusion in terms and definitions impact either intern physician communications or understanding of manufacturers' and engineers' instructions and limitations when using devices (M. Cecconi).

The International Bureau of Weights and Measures defines metrology as the science of measurement, embracing both experimental and theoretical determinations at any level of uncertainty in any field of science and technology.

IMPORTANT CONCEPTS IN METROLOGY

The Metrological list of terms found in the Joint Committee for Guides in Metrology is divided into 5 main headings: Quantities and Units, Measurements, Devices for Measurements, Properties of Measuring Devices and Measuring Standards.

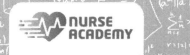

UNITS OF MEASUREMENT

The most commonly used prefixes that apply to clinical practice are:

Mega – this prefix indicates millions. Benzylpenicillin, a penicillin antibiotic that is administered by injection, is available in vials containing one mega unit.

Milli – this prefix indicates a thousandth of a unit. One milligram is one-thousandth of a gram. Aciclovir dispersible tablets, used to treat shingles, contain 800 milligrams.

Micro – this prefix indicates a millionth of a unit. One microgram is one-millionth of a gram. (There are one thousand micrograms in one milligram and one thousand milligrams in one gram. One thousand multiplied by one thousand equals one million.)Glyceryl triturate, taken to relieve angina, is available in tablets containing 500 micrograms.

Nano – this prefix indicates a thousand-millionth of a unit. This is extremely small and rarely used in clinical practice

VOLUME

Volume is measured in liters or subunits of a liter, milliliters. 1000 milliliters is equal to one liter. The standard abbreviation for liter is L and the abbreviation for milliliter is ml.

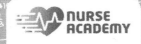

WEIGHT

KILOGRAMS

The SI unit of weight is the kilogram, which can be subdivided into smaller units several times. Kilograms are useful when measuring large items like body weight, but when measuring small amounts of drugs, alternative units of measurement are needed. The unit smaller than one kilogram is a gram, and 1000 grams equal one kilogram.

$$1,000 \, g = 1 \, kilogram \, (kg)$$

GRAMS AND MILLIGRAMS

Grams are widely used within clinical practice in drug administration. Grams can be divided into smaller units called milligrams; there are 1000 milligrams in one gram. Two 500 milligram paracetamol tablets are the equivalent of one gram. The correct abbreviation of milligram is 'mg'. Morphine is an opioid analgesic frequently used to control severe pain; it can be injected (intramuscularly, intravenously, and subcutaneously) and administered orally. As an oral solution, it is available in several different strengths. One of these contains 2 mg in 1 ml, therefore in 5 ml there are 10 mg.

$$1,000 \, mg = 1 \, gram \, (g)$$
$$1,000 \, mcg = 1 \, mg$$

MICROGRAMS

Milligrams can also be divided into smaller units called micrograms. There are 1000 micrograms in one milligram. Converting milligrams to micrograms follows the same rule as when converting kilograms to grams and grams to milligrams.

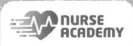

PRESSURE

The commonly used unit for the measurement of blood pressure in clinical practice in the UK is millimeters of mercury, which has the abbreviation 'mmHg'. Capital letters aren't routinely used as abbreviations for units of measurement, but Hg is the international symbol for the element mercury. You will see this displayed on sphygmomanometers used to measure and record a patient's blood pressure.

There is also an SI unit for pressure called the Pascal (abbreviation Pa), which is named after the French physicist and mathematician Blaise Pascal (1623–1662). The Pascal is a small unit, so you are more likely to see it referred to using the prefix kilo, as kilopascal (kPa).

QUANTITIES AND UNITS

Quantities are properties of a phenomenon, body, or substance, attributed to a magnitude that can be expressed as a number and a reference. A quantity is a scalar. A reference can be a measurement unit, a measurement procedure, a reference material, or a combination of such. A quantity is characterized by a dimension, a unit, and a value.

MEASUREMENT

This is the process of experimentally obtaining values that can be attributed to quantity. The true value of a quantity is unique at a specific time and is always

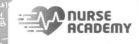

unknown. The result is generally expressed as a single measured quantity and a measurement uncertainty. A measurement method is based on a principle; a physical, chemical, or biological phenomenon serving as the basis of measurement.

MEASUREMENT ACCURACY

This is the closeness of agreement between a measured quantity value and a true quantity value of the measured. The concept of accuracy is a quality and is not given a numerical value. A measurement is said to be more accurate when it offers a smaller measurement error. Therefore, a measurement error is qualifying a single measurement.

MEASUREMENT TRUENESS

This is the closeness of agreement between the average of an infinite number of replicate measured quantity values and the true or a reference quantity value. The concept of trueness is a quality and is not given a numerical value. Measurement trueness is inversely related to systematic measurement error but not to random measurement error.

MEASUREMENT PRECISION

This is the closeness of agreement between measured quantity values obtained by replicate measurements on the same or similar objects under specified conditions.

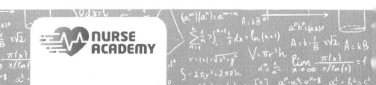

Measurement precision is related to random measurement error and is usually expressed numerically by measures of imprecision.

ROMAN NUMERALS

Roman numerals are commonly used when writing prescriptions despite not being recommended for practice. Here, letters are used to indicate numbers.

Roman Numeral	Ordinary Number
I (or i)	1
II (or ii)	2
III (or iii)	3
IV (or iv)	4
V (or v)	5
VI (or vi)	6
VII (or vii)	7
VIII (or viii)	8
IX (or ix)	9
X (or x)	10
L (or l)	50

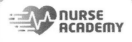

C (or c)	100
D (or d)	500
M (or m)	1,000

HOW TO READ ROMAN NUMERALS

There are rules to reading Roman numerals whether they are in capital letters or small letters. The position of one letter in relation to the other is important and determines the value of the numeral. These are some of the rules that have to be adhered to.

Roman and Numerals	
½ = ss	5 = v
1 = I or i	10 = x
2 = II or ii	15 = xv
3 = III or iii	19 = xix [10 + (10-1)] or xix
4 = IV or iv (i before v = 5-1) or iv	20 = xx

- When you repeat a Roman numeral twice, it doubles its value; the same happens when you repeat it three times: it triples its value.
- The letter I is usually repeated up to three times while V is written once only.

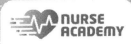

- When a smaller Roman numeral is placed after a larger one, add the two together.

- Subtract the smaller numeral from the larger one when a smaller Roman numeral is placed before a larger one.

- Apply the subtraction rule, then add when a Roman numeral of a smaller value comes between two larger values.

FRACTIONS AND DECIMALS

Fractions and decimals are helpful since they are involved in most calculations. Calculating decimals through multiplication and division through fractions is important.

FRACTIONS

A fraction is part of a whole number or one number divided by another.

Example: 2/5 is a fraction and means 2 parts of 5 where 5 is a whole value.

The value above the 'line' is called the numerator and it indicates the number of parts of the whole value that is being used.

The value below the 'line' is called the denominator and it indicates the number of parts into which the whole is divided.

Therefore, in the example, the whole has been divided into 5 equal parts.

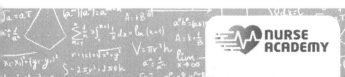

Simplifying Fractions

When not using a calculator, it is easier to work with simplified fractions to their lowest terms. To simplify a fraction, choose any number that divides exactly into the numerator and the denominator.

When a fraction is no longer possible to divide the numerator and denominator by the same number, it is considered to have been reduced to its lowest terms.

Cancellation is the process of converting or reducing fractions to their simplest form.

Note: Whatever happens to the top line, must happen to the bottom line. Simplifying a fraction to its lowest terms does not change the value of the fraction.

DECIMALS

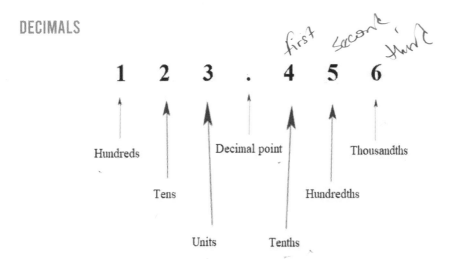

Decimals describe the 'tenths' value of a number, in terms of 10. A decimal number consists of a decimal point and numbers both to the left and right of that decimal

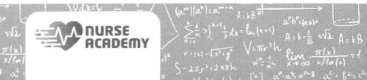

point. The numbers to the left of the decimal point are greater than one. Numbers to the right of the decimal point are less than one

RULES

When making drug calculations, it is vital that you work with the same units. If your units don't match, it is advisable to first convert them to achieve this. i.e., mg or mcg but not both units at the same time.

The first rule to watch is to ensure that the administered dose is reasonable from the drug calculation you have achieved, thus; a 600 g dose of antibiotics or a 20-tablet dose of a Furosemide are both likely to be wrong. This way, if you are not certain of your calculations, especially on complex dose calculations, get some-one to help check the results.

- Place the whole Number over 1 when writing in a fraction

  3 tablets = 3/1

  5 mgs = 5/1

- Double-check your answer when moving a decimal to the right or left of Zero. Whole Number to the Left (Units, Tens, Hundreds, thousands, Ten-thousands). Decimal to the Right (Tenths, Hundredths, Thousandths, Ten-thousandths).

- Move a decimal point two places to the right when changing a decimal point to a percentage

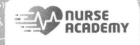

0.1 = 10%, 0.01 = 0.1%

- To obtain the percentage, multiply a fraction by 100

  ½ × 100/1 = 50%

  1/5 × 100/1 = 20%

- Divide the percentage by a denominator of 100 when changing a percent to a fraction

  50% = 50/100

  500/2% = 500/2 × 1/100 = 5/2

- Reverse the Divisor and multiply with the percent that are mixed fractions

- Change the percentage to a decimal and multiply by the whole number when calculating the percentage of a whole number

  100% of 50 = 1.00 × 50 = 50.0

  5% of 25 = 0.05 × 25 = 1.25

- Review Roman Numerals - Medications are sometimes ordered using Roman numerals

  Tylenol X grains q6h orally

- Round down numbers <5 and up for numbers =/>5

  99.96 = 100.0

  1.2 = 1.0

Note: Consider the kind of medication you are administering. Some can be given in tenths or hundredths.

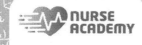

THE INTERNATIONAL METRIC DECIMAL MEASUREMENT SYSTEM

There are three different types of measurements in medications:

Type	Number	Solids	Liquids
Apothecary	Whole numbers and fractions before unit Ex: 1½ T	Teaspoons (tsp, t) Tablespoons (Tbs, T) Pounds (lb)	Drop (gtt) Ounce (oz) Cup (c) Pint (pt) Quart (qt) Glass
Household	Whole numbers, fractions, and Roman numerals after unit Ex: gr 15 ½	Grains (gr) Drams (dr or 3)	Minum (m) Fluid Dram (dr or 3)
Metric	Whole numbers and decimals before unit (always put a 0 in front of the decimal) Ex: 0.15 Ml	Grams (g) Meter (m)	Liters (L)

Remember, Consider the unit of the final answer when two system-to-system conversion factors exist.

Example:

Use the gr 1 = 60 mg conversion factor if it is necessary for the drug dosage problem to convert a dosage from grains to mg.

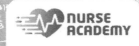

APPROXIMATE CONVERSION FACTORS

SOLID CONVERSIONS

gr 1 = 60 mg

gr 15 = 1 g

2.54 cm = 1 in

2.2 lb = 1 kg

FLUID CONVERSIONS

1 oz = dr 8 or 38

m 15 = 1 mL = 1 cc

4 mL = fluid dr 1 = 31

15 mL = 3 t = 1 T

30 mL = 1 oz

EXTENDED CONVERSIONS

1 kg = 1000 g = 2.2 lbs

1 L = 1000 mL = 33 1/3 oz = 200 t = 66 2/3 T = 3250

VISUAL CONVERSIONS "THE GRAIN CLOCK"

Convert grains to mg:

gr 1 = 60 mg

1 hour = 60 min

gr ¾ = 45 mg

¾ hour = 45 min

gr ¼ = 15 mg

¼ hour = 15 min

gr ½ = 30 mg

½ hour = 30 min

INCHES TO CENTIMETERS

1 inch = 2.54 cm

CONVERSION BETWEEN UNITS

USING A ONE-CONVERSION FACTOR

When converting from one unit to another, begin with the unit assigned. The next step is to find a conversion factor relating the unit assigned to the unit needed. Multiply the unit assigned by the converted factor. This calculation results in a new unit.

Example:

Convert 120 mg to gr_____.

Consider a conversion factor that relates to mg and gr. 60 mg = gr

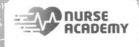

- Set up the multiplication equation.
- Remember, when using the conversion: 120 mg • gr 1 = gr
- Factor, place the needed unit on top: 60 mg
- Solve the equation.

Begin by cancelling mg units:

$$\frac{120 \text{ mg} \bullet \text{gr } 1}{60 \text{ mg}} = \text{gr} \_\_\_\_\_$$

Solve the equation: 120 • gr 1 ÷ 60 = gr 2

Hence: 120 mg = gr 2

USE OF MULTIPLE CONVERSION

Proceed through another unit to obtain the unit needed when a conversion factor

for the two units does not exist.

Example: TSP

Convert 1 T to _____oz.

Find a conversion factor that relates tablespoons to ounces. From the list, there

is no conversion factor relating to tablespoons and ounces.

Hence, two conversion factors are needed: 1 T = 15 mL and 30 mL = 1 oz.

Set up the equations:

$$\frac{1 \text{ T} \bullet 15 \text{ mL}}{1 \text{ T}} = \_15\_ \text{ mL} \qquad \frac{\_\_\_\_\_ \text{ mL} \bullet 1 \text{ oz}}{30 \text{ mL}} = \_\_\_\_\_\text{oz}$$

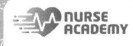

Solve the equations:

1T• 15 mL ÷ 1T

T= 15 mL

15 mL• 1 oz ÷ 30 mL= 0.5 oz

Therefore: 1 T = 0.5 oz

CONVERTING BETWEEN METRIC UNITS

When converting between metric units, move the decimal place.

Symbol	k	H	D	b	d	c	m t	mc
Name	kilo	Hector	Deca	"base"	deci	centi	milli	micro
Ex.	kg	Hg	Dg	gram	dg	cg	mg	mcg

There are three decimal places between m and mc, which is often forgotten.

Using the chat, conversions between metric units involves locating the starting place then sliding the decimal to the desired unit and adding zeros as required or needed.

Example 2:

$$\frac{1\ g}{1,000\ mg}$$

X →

Convert 25.3 g to _25,300_ mg

The given unit is in grams; start at "b".

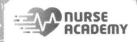

The ending place is m; slide the decimal from "b" to "m".

-- h D b d c m . . mc

$1,000 \text{ mg} = 1 \text{ g}$

25.3 → 25. 3 0 0. → 25,300 mg Slide 3 decimal places to the right

Hence: 25.3 g = 25,300 mg

$1 \text{ mg} = 1,000 \text{ mcg}$

Example 3:

Convert 300 mcg to __0.3__ mg

$\dfrac{300 \text{ mcg}}{1} \cdot \dfrac{1 \text{ mg}}{1,000 \text{ mcg}} = \dfrac{300}{1000}$

The given unit is mc; start at "mc".

The ending place is m; slide the decimal from "mc" to "m".

k h D b d c m . . mc

300 → 3 0 0. → 0.300 mg Slide decimal 3 places to left (mc to m)

Hence: 300 mcg = 0.300 mg

CALCULATING DRUG DOSAGES

There are several different methods that can be used during drug calculation. We will review this in the next chapter. But first, let's identify the four methods that should be used:

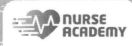

1. Ratio (Rainbow) Method

2. Proportion Method

3. Formula Method

4. Dimensional Analysis

These methods work as well as each other, however, once a student decides which method they are comfortable with, they should stick with that method.

RATIO:

- Step one: Set up ratios.

- Step two: Multiply means and extremes

- Step three: Solve for "x" algebraically.

PROPORTION:

- Step one: Set up proportions

- Step two: Cross multiply

- Step three: Solve for "x" algebraically

FORMULA:

(D • Q) / H = answer

$$\frac{D \text{ (dose ordered)} \cdot Q \text{ (unit quantity)}}{H \text{ (Dose on hand)}} = \text{answer}$$

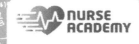

DIMENSIONAL ANALYSIS:

When calculating the quantity of medication needed for a patient, and the strength of medication is already known, use the drug calculation formula.

Example:

If the doctor orders 20 mg of Benadryl, and 10 mg tablets are available, how many tablets should be given to the patient?

$$\frac{20 \text{ mg}}{10 \text{ mg}} = 2 \text{ tablets}$$

USING RATIO (RAINBOW) METHOD

10 mg = 1 tablet, we need 20 mg in an unknown number of tablets.

Step one: Set up ratios

10 mg : 1 tab = 20 mg : x tab

Note: On both sides of the equation, mg comes first, then tablets. This is very important.

Here, it doesn't matter which unit comes first, as long as units are in the same order on both sides of the equal "=" sign.

Step two: Multiply means and extremes

10 mg • x tab = 1 tab • 20 mg

Step three: Solve for "x" algebraically

$$x \text{ tab} = \frac{1 \text{ tab} \cdot 20}{10 \text{ mg}}$$

x = 2 tablets

USING PROPORTION METHOD

- Set up proportions:

$$\frac{10 \text{ mg}}{1 \text{ tab}} = \frac{20 \text{ mg}}{x \text{ tab}}$$

- Cross multiply:

  10 mg • x tab = 20 mg • 1 tab

- Solve for "x" algebraically

$$x \text{ tab} = \frac{20 \cancel{\text{ mg}} \cdot 1 \text{ tab}}{10 \cancel{\text{ mg}}}$$

x = 2 tablets

USING FORMULA METHOD

(D • Q) / H = answer

So:

$$\frac{20 \text{ mg} \cdot 1 \text{ tab}}{10 \text{ mg}} = 2 \text{ tablets}$$

Hence: the patient is given 2 tablets.

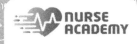

IMPORTANT FORMULAS FOR CALCULATING

DRUG CALCULATION PROBLEMS

CALCULATING BSA (M²):

$$\frac{Lb \times in}{3131} \quad or \quad \frac{kg \times cm}{3600}$$ Round to hundredths place after taking the square root

Example:

A patient weighs 140 lb and is 62 inches tall, find the BSA.

$$\frac{140\ lb \times 62\ in}{3,131}$$

$140 \times 62 = 8,680$

$8,680 \div 3131 = 2.77$

$\sqrt{2.77} = 1.66\ m^2$

- Round to hundredths place
- Answer is always in m^2

FINDING A CHILD'S DOSAGE USING AN ADULT DOSAGE:

$$\frac{Child's\ BSA}{1.7\ m^2} \times Adult\ Dosage = Child's\ Dosage$$

Example:

The normal adult dosage of a medication is 150 mg. The child weighs 32 kg and is 120 cm tall. Calculate the medication that should be given to the child?

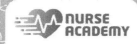

Find the child's BSA:

$$\frac{32 \text{ kg} \times 120 \text{ cm}}{3,600} = 1.0666$$

$$\sqrt{1.0666\ldots} = 1.032792\ldots \text{ m}^2 = 1.03 \text{ m}^2$$

- Round to hundredths place

Use the child's dosage formula:

$$\underline{1.03 \text{ m}^2} \times 150 \text{ mg} = 90.88 \text{ mg}$$

- Round to hundredths place

1.7 m^2

DETERMINING FLOW RATE IN ML/H:

$$\frac{\text{Total mL ordered}}{\text{Total hours ordered}} = \frac{\text{mL}}{\text{h}} \text{ (must round to a whole number)}$$

Example:

Calculate the flow rate for an IV of 1,820 mL Normal Saline IV to infuse in 15 h by controller.

$$\frac{1,820 \text{ mL}}{15 \text{h}} =$$

Flow rate = $\left(\underline{121} \right)$ mL/h

1,820 mL = 121.33 mL/h = 121 mL/h

- Round to nearest whole number

15 h

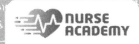

CALCULATING FLOW RATE IN GTT/MIN:

$$\frac{\text{Volume (mL)} \cdot \text{drop factor (gtt/mL)}}{\text{Time (min)}} = \text{Rate (gtt/min)}$$

CALCULATING HEPARIN DOSAGES:

Order: D5W

$$\frac{40{,}000 \text{ U}}{1{,}000 \text{ mL}} = \frac{x \text{ U}}{40 \text{ mL}} \quad \text{Cross multiply}$$

x U • 1,000 mL = 40,000 U • 40 mL

Then divide by 1000 mL

$$\frac{40{,}000\text{U} \cdot 40 \text{ mL}}{1{,}000 \text{ mL}} = \frac{1{,}600{,}000 \text{ U}}{1000} = 1600 \text{ U/hr}$$

Heparin 40,000 U in 1,000 mL D5W to infuse at 40 mL/h. What is the hourly heparin dosage?

Calculate the number of units there are in 40 mL.

CONVERTING FROM ºF TO ºC OR ºC TO ºF:

- Carry to hundredths and round to tenths

$$ºF = 1.8 \cdot (ºC) + 32$$

$$ºC = \frac{ºF - 32}{1.8}$$

FORMULAS AND SOLUTIONS

Inadequate experience and the slightest errors in math calculations are still a major source of drug errors.

Nursing competence in drug calculations has been a cause for concern (Duffin, 2000; Coombes, 2000). According to Hutton, 1998, a degree of 'de-skilling' has resulted from the increasing user-friendliness of drug preparations and widespread use of electronic drip counters.

According to her studies, reports indicated that most students could not perform calculations like long divisions and fractions without using calculators as they used them at school. An extensive debate on calculator use, Hutton (1998) argues that calculators are usually available in areas where calculations are complex, and that their use should be encouraged.

The opinion of the Nursing and Midwifery Council is that nurses should not rely too heavily on calculators, stating that administration of medicines (UKCC, 2000) and use of calculators 'should not act as a substitute for arithmetical knowledge and skill.' To develop calculation skills, one has to understand decimals to make conversion easier. When using long division, it is essential to get it the right way.

Most students have interpreted drug calculations as impossible and difficult unless broken down into small steps. This topic highlights the commonly used drug calculations and how mistakes can happen.

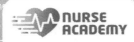

FORMULA 1

When the dose you want is not a complete vial.

For example:

- Prescription states 100mg
- You have an ampoule of 500mg in 4ml

The Right Volume for the Right Dose

If you have a vial of 250mg in 2ml, and you need 100mg, it can appear to be a doubtful calculation. First, start by finding out what volume contains 1mg (2/250) and then multiply it by the number of mg you want (100).

The famous nursing equation is the easy way to remember this: 'What you want, over what you have, multiplied by what is in'.

In this case: 100mg x 2ml / 250mg = 0.8 ml

Here, the common error would be to calculate the inverted, and divide what you have by what you want. This automatically gives the wrong answer.

Converting Units

All measurements in any equation must be in the same units. For weights, the unit changes every thousand.

For example, you need 1000 micrograms (mcg) to make 1 milligram (mg) and 1000 milligrams to make one gram (g) (Box 2).

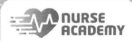

FORMULA 2

These include the infusion rate calculations.

Example:

- Prescription states 30 mg/hour
- You have a bag containing 250mg in 50ml

What Is the Rate That You Set the Pump In (ml/hr)?

This is almost similar to Formula 1. Once you have worked out the volume con-taining the amount of drug you need, then you can set the pump to give that amount per hour.

In this case, work out how many ml contain ONE mg of the drug.

Using the WIG equation:

30 x 50 / 250 = 6ml

Hence, the calculation indicates that for 30mg per hour, the infusion pump rate would need to be set at 6ml per hour.

This calculation is easy and straightforward when the rate you want (30mg/hour) and the amount of the drug in the bag (250mg) are both in the same units (mg).

On the other hand, if the infusion stated that 600 micrograms be infused each hour, this would need to be converted into mg before the infusion rate was cal-culated, that is, 600 micrograms = 0.6mg.

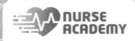

The equation for infusion rate:

Dose stated in prescription (mg.hr) multiplied by volume in the syringe (in ml) divided by the volume in the syringe (in ml)

FORMULA 3

When the infusion rate is required, but the dose is 'mg per kg'.

Example:

- Prescription states 0.5mg/kg/hour
- You have a bag of 250mg in 50ml
- Your patient weighs 70kg

For this calculation, use the WIG equation as above, but with an extra step to work out the 'what you want'.

Start by converting the mg per kg into total mg by multiplying it by the patient's weight.

For someone weighing 70kg, 0.5mg per kg is the same as 35mg. Once you have calculated this, the infusion rate can be worked out as in Formula 2.

In this case:

0.5mg/kg/hr x 70kg x 50ml / 250mg = 7ml/hr

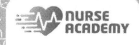

FORMULA 4

When the infusion rate is needed and the dose is in mg/kg/min

Example:

- Prescription states 0.5mg/kg/min
- You have a syringe of 250mg in 50ml
- Your patient weighs 70kg

Like before, calculate what you want by multiplying the amount per kg by the patient's weight.

0.5mg x 70kg = 35mg

Note, the prescription requires the rate per minute. The pump requires that the rate be set in ml per hour, therefore convert the rate per minute before the equation can be completed, by multiplying 35 by 60; that is, 35mg/min (35 milligrams per minute) is converted to 2100mg/hr (2100 milligrams per hour).

From this point, use Formula 2 to find the infusion rate, which will be 420ml/hr.

2100 x 50 / 250mg = 420ml/hr

FORMULA 5

When the infusion rate is required and the dose is in mcg/kg/min.

Example:

- Prescription states 3 micrograms (mcg)/kg/min

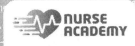

- You have a syringe of 100mg in 50ml
- Your patient weighs 70kg

Here what you want is calculated by multiplying the amount per kg by the patient's weight:

3mcg/kg for a 70kg person is 210mcg

Convert the prescription rate to rate per hour.

210mcg/min = 12 600mcg/hr

The prescription is in mcg, while you have ml in your syringe. To have the two in the same unit, convert one to the other:

mcg to mg. 12 600mcg/hr is the same as 12.6mg/hr.

The calculation becomes:

12.6 x 50 / 100 = 6.3ml/hr

PROPORTIONS

There are various methods used to calculate dosages. 'Ratio and proportion' and use of a formula' are some of the most used ones.

Students can choose methods from the various ones we will review and which they will find convenient and logical to use.

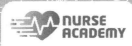

PROPORTION IN DOSAGE CALCULATION

It is important to recall that the use of proportion may produce a single quantity answer and that after comparing two ratios.

Say you had a medication of dosage strength 50 mg per 1 Ml. and a dosage strength of 25mg is prescribed, the proportion may be used to determine how many milliliters to administer.

When setting up a proportion using the fraction format to calculate dosages, the known ratio is what you get, and often stated first (placed on the left side of the proportion). What is ordered to be prescribed is the unknown.

Example 1

$$\frac{50 \text{ mg}}{1 \text{ mL}} = \frac{25 \text{ mg}}{x \text{ mL}}$$
$$\text{(known)} \qquad \text{(unknown)}$$

The information on the medication label is stated first when writing the ratio and proportion using the colons, and the unknown ratio is stated second.

$$\frac{50x}{50} = \frac{25}{50}$$

x = 0.5 mL

Note that the known is stated as the first fraction and the unknown as the second. Solve by cross multiplication when stated in fraction format.

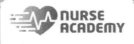

Or:

50x = product of extremes

25 = product of means

50x = 25 is the equation

$$\frac{50x}{50} = \frac{25}{50}$$ (Divide both sides by 50, the number in front of x.)

x= 0.5 mL

Remember it is essential to state the units of measure in the same sequence:

$$\frac{mg}{mL} = \frac{mg}{mL}$$

or mg : mL = mg : mL.

Example 2

Prescribe: 40 mg p.o. of a medication.

Available: 20 mg tablets. Calculate the number of tablets to be administered

$$\frac{20 \text{ mg}}{1 \text{ tab}} = \frac{40 \text{ mg}}{x \text{ tab}}$$
$$\quad\text{(known)} \qquad\quad \text{(unknown)}$$

$$\frac{20x}{20} = \frac{40}{20}$$

x = 2 tabs

Or:

$$\frac{20 \text{ mg} : 1 \text{ tab}}{\text{(known)}} = \frac{40 \text{ mg} : x \text{ tab}}{\text{(unknown)}}$$

$$\frac{20x}{20} = \frac{40}{20}$$

x = 2 tabs

Example 3

Order 1 g p.o. of an antibiotic 500 mg capsules available. Find the number of capsules to be prescribed.

Note that the ordered dosage is in a different unit from what is available. Start by changing the units of measure so they are the same and set up the problem and calculate the dosage to be given. The conversion is within the same metric.

Grams are converted to milligrams by using the equivalent 1,000 mg = 1 g. After making the conversion, the ratio is stated as follows:

$$\frac{500 \text{ mg}}{1 \text{ cap}} = \frac{1{,}000 \text{ mg}}{x \text{ caps}}$$
(known)   (unknown)

x = 2 caps

Or:

$$\frac{500 \text{ mg} : 1 \text{ cap}}{\text{(known)}} = \frac{1{,}000 \text{ mg} : x \text{ caps}}{\text{(unknown)}}$$

x = 2 caps

Alternatively, convert milligrams to grams. This will convert 500 mg to grams by using the same equivalent: 1,000 mg = 1 g.

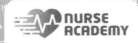

However, you should know that decimals are common when measures are changed from smaller to larger in the metric system:

500 mg = 0.5 g.

Despite the fact that converting the milligrams to grams would provide the same result, calculation errors are often a result of conversions that produce decimals, hence, avoid conversions that require their use. It is often recommended to convert the stated measure on the medication label. Doing this repeatedly will prevent confusion.

Determining whether an answer is logical is necessary for the calculation of a medication.

It is important to:

- Ensure that all terms are in the same unit and metrics before calculating. If not, do a conversion before calculating dosage.
- Conversions can be made by converting what is ordered to the units in which the medication is available when the conversion of units is needed. This can also be done by changing what is available to the units in which the medication is ordered. Be consistent with how you make conversions - convert what is ordered to the same unit and system of measure you have the medication available in.
- Start with the known when stating ratios. The known ratio is the available information obtained from the medication label.

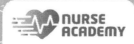

- The unknown ratio is the dosage desired and is stated second.
- Indicate the terms of the ratios in the proportion, including *x*.
- Make a mental estimate of the approximate and reasonable answer before calculating the dosage.
- Indicate the value you obtain for *x* (e.g., mL, tabs). Countercheck the label for *x* by referring to the label of *x* in the original ratio and proportion; this should match.
- A proportion can be stated in a horizontal way using colons or as a fraction.
- Countercheck all work. Ensure consistency in stating ratios and conversions.

An error in the setup of the ratio and proportion can cause an error in calculation. Intravenous fluids can be dangerous to children, it is advisable that wherever possible, oral rehydration solution orally or via nasogastric way be used.

MAINTENANCE FLUIDS IN CHILDREN

FLUID REQUIREMENTS

Total daily fluid requirements (over 24 hours)	
1st 10kg of bodyweight	100ml/kg/day

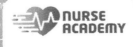

2nd 10kg of bodyweight	50ml/kg/day
Remainder of bodyweight	20ml/kg/day

Rate (ml/h) = total daily requirement ÷ 24

Example:

A child with 27kg maintenance requirements would be:

Daily requirement:

1st 10kg = 100ml/kg/day = 1000ml

2nd 10kg = 50ml/kg/day = 500ml

Rest (i.e., 7kg) = 20ml/kg/day = 140ml

TOTAL = 1640ml/day

Rate = 1640 ÷ 24 = <u>68ml/hour</u>

ELECTROLYTE REQUIREMENTS

Sodium = 2-4mmol/kg/day (but this 'requirement' of sodium is ignored because it was based on a study involving healthy, overweight American children with high-salt diets; 0.9% saline+5% dextrose has now been proven to be the safest maintenance fluid in hospitalized children)

Potassium = 1-2mmol/kg/day (but the fluid type below (500ml bag with 10mmol KCl) at the rate above will give the right amount of potassium in most cases)

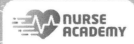

The fluid type that is usually used for maintenance is 500ml 0.9% saline + 5% dextrose with 10mmol KCl (all in the same bag) – there are different concentrations of potassium available if required

MAINTENANCE FLUIDS IN NEONATES

FLUID REQUIREMENTS

Day 1: 60ml/kg/day

Day 2: 90ml/kg/day

Day 3: 120ml/kg/day

Day 4 and after: 150ml/kg/d

The formula above still applies – work out their total daily requirement first, then divide by 24 to get the hourly infusion rate.

Notes:

- Small or premature infants require more fluids due to higher insensible losses (extra 20ml/kg/day if <1.5kg, extra 40ml/kg/day if <1kg)
- If the baby weighs less than their birth weight, use the birth weight to calculate their fluid requirement
- If the baby is: <1kg measure electrolytes 8-12 hourly for 3-4 days, then daily; <1.5kg 12 hourly for 3-4 days then daily; >1.5kg daily.

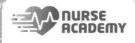

- Weigh all babies daily

ELECTROLYTE REQUIREMENTS

These are very important in neonates and are added to the bag manually. Electrolyte requirements depend on their electrolyte results, but average requirements are:

Sodium = 3mmol/kg/day (range 2-4mmol/kg/day; 4mmol/kg/day if preterm)

Potassium = 2mmol/kg/day (range 1-3mmol/kg/day)

Note: only start adding sodium and potassium once post-natal diuresis starts to occur (and hence levels start to decline) on day 2-3

The only fluid type used for maintenance should be 500ml 10% dextrose with personalized amounts of sodium and potassium added.

The calculation of electrolyte additives can be complex because you need to calculate the concentration of electrolytes needed to be added to 500ml to give their requirements over 24 hours.

Taking into account that the 500ml may run over more/less than 24 hours, work out the total daily fluid requirement, calculate the total daily sodium and potassium requirement, and because the fluid comes in 500ml bags, the additives required can be calculated by:

Total days the bag will run over = 500ml ÷ daily fluid requirement

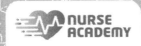

Electrolyte additive required = total days the bag will run over x daily electrolyte requirement Work it out for sodium and potassium separately.

EXISTING DEHYDRATION CORRECTION

How to estimate the severity of dehydration and fluid deficit from the clinical features present			
Dehydration severity	Deficit (ml/kg)	Clinical features	Management
Mild	50ml/kg (5% body weight)	Slightly dry mucus membranes, increased thirst, slightly decreased urine output	Oral/NG rehydration solution (1-1.5x maintenance) OR: IV maintenance
Moderate	100ml/kg (10% body weight)	Dry mucus membranes, <u>tachycardia</u>, reduced urine output, loss of skin turgor, sunken eyes/fontanelle	IV bolus OR: NG fluids at 25ml/kg/h for first 4 hours; oral rehydration solution
Severe	150ml/kg (15% body weight)	As in moderate but also: pronounced <u>tachycardia</u>, weak pulse, hypotension, delayed capillary refill, mottled skin/cyanosis, dyspnoea	IV bolus (may need multiple)

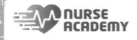

A fluid bolus of 10-20ml/kg 0.9% saline may be given STAT to replace a significant fluid deficit. Only moderate-severe dehydration should be corrected with an IV fluid bolus (because a fluid bolus is not without risk in children).

The aim of a bolus is to restore blood pressure and perfusion. Boluses should be used to reduce moderate/severe dehydration to a deficit of ~80ml/kg (8% body weight) – below which blood pressure and perfusion are adequate.

e.g., in moderate dehydration, a 20ml/kg bolus will reduce a 100ml/kg deficit to an 80ml/kg deficit

In severe dehydration, repeat 20ml/kg boluses may be required.

Mild dehydration, or the remaining deficit, should be corrected with oral or NG rehydration solution, or by IV fluids aiming to correct the deficit <u>over 24-48 hours</u> (in addition to normal maintenance if that is also required).

However, unless the patient is strictly nil by mouth, the maintenance rate is usually adequate, because they will start drinking again when they've 'turned corner.'

Oral rehydration solution fluid challenge (for mild-moderate gastroenteritis) =

1-2ml/kg of oral rehydration solution every 10 minutes

Give parents a chart to fill in

20ml/kg of oral fluid in 2 hours = adequate (if not, the child may need admission)

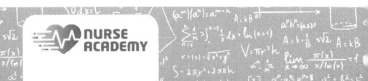

ONGOING LOSSES CORRECTION

Estimate the rate of loss and replace at the same rate. If you are replacing a particular loss that is being measured, you can prescribe the fluid as "ml for ml of stoma loss". The type of fluid depends on the fluid lost. Extracellular fluid losses are most similar to 500ml 0.9% saline with 13.5mmol KCl. Fever = same type of fluids as normal maintenance fluids (500ml 0.9% saline+5% dextrose with 10mmol KCl). If the patient is on maintenance fluids and requires extra to correct losses/deficit you can quantify extra fluids as 'maintenance + 5/10/15%'

Note: Only in special situations, for hypo/hypernatraemia, correct the fluid deficit slowly unless the patient is shocked.

INTRAVENOUS INFUSION

Often, nurses get intimidated by calculations they have to face every other day in their practice. Patient safety relies entirely on the medics' ability to calculate correct medications in a timely manner. This topic provides a simple method for accurate computation using basic calculations.

With the programmable I.V. pumps used in many clinical settings, nurses need to verify the correct dosage by calculation once during the shift and often if a medication is being titrated or changed. Another available resource in many practice settings is the pharmacy.

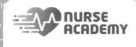

Pharmacists are knowledgeable about medications and have unparalleled proficiency with drug calculations. Knowing the therapeutic dosage for the desired effect is as important as knowing the correct calculations for the drug.

Example:

Dopamine at doses of 3 to 5 mcg/kg/minute gives a gentle dilatation of the renal arteries, increasing urine output with no effect on BP. At higher doses (up to 20 mcg/kg/minute), dopamine is used for BP support.

Identify the medication and what effect you're attempting to achieve, and the maximum recommended safe infusion dosage.

Try the following methods for calculating. Patient medication safety is a goal that all practitioners have in common and it all starts with doing the math!

BASIC CALCULATIONS

The universal formula is:

$$\frac{D\,(\text{desired amount})}{H\,(\text{amount on hand})} \times V\,(\text{volume}) = \text{Dose}$$

Administer heparin 5,000 units I.V. push. Available is heparin 10,000 units/mL. calculate the ml you will need to administer a 5,000-unit dose

$$\frac{5{,}000\ \text{units}\,(D)}{10{,}000\ \text{units}\,(H)} \times 1\ \text{mL}\,(V) = X$$

Answer: X = 0.5 mL

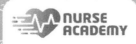

CALCULATIONS IN MCG/MINUTE

Follow the steps below to administer a patient's accurate drug dosage.

- Find out what's in the I.V. bottle (that is, the drug concentration or the number of mL of fluid).
- Determine the units your drug is measured in (units/hour, mg/hour, or mcg/kg/minute).
- Find out the patient's weight in kg if your calculation is weight-based.

QUICK REFERENCE: UNIVERSAL FORMULAS

Basic dosage calculation:

$$\frac{D \text{ (desired amount)}}{H \text{ (amount on hand)}} \times V \text{ (volume)} = Dose$$

I.V. drips in mcg/minute

$$\frac{mg}{mL} \rightarrow \frac{1{,}000 \text{ mcg}}{1 \text{ mg}} \rightarrow \frac{mL}{1 \text{ hour}} \rightarrow \frac{1 \text{ hour}}{60 \text{ minutes}} = mcg/minute$$

($\div$ by kg to get mcg/kg/minute)

Use the universal formula and then divide your final answer by the patient's weight in kg to arrive at mcg/kg/minute.

Example:

Dopamine is infusing. The bottle states dopamine 800 mg, and it's mixed in 500 mL of D$_5$W. The I.V. pump in your patient's room is set at 15 mL, and the patient

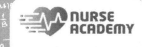

weighs 60 kg (60,000 g). At how many mcg/kg/minutes is the patient's dopamine infusing?

$$\frac{800 \text{ mg}}{500 \text{ mL}} \rightarrow \frac{1,000 \text{ mcg}}{1 \text{ mg}} \rightarrow \frac{15 \text{ mL}}{1 \text{ hour}} \rightarrow \frac{1 \text{ hour}}{60 \text{ minutes}} \div 60 \text{ kg} = X$$

Answer: X = 6.7 mcg/kg/minute

Example:

Dobutamine 200 mg in 250 mL of D$_5$W is ordered to run at 5 mcg/kg/minute. At how many mL/hour will you set the pump?

$$\frac{200 \text{ mg}}{250 \text{ mL}} \rightarrow \frac{1,000 \text{ mcg}}{1 \text{ mg}} \rightarrow \frac{X}{1 \text{ hour}} \rightarrow \frac{1 \text{ hour}}{60 \text{ minutes}} \div 60 \text{kg} = 5 \text{ mcg/kg/min}$$

Answer: X = 22.5 mL/hour

I.V. drips in units/hour

To arrive at units/hour, the universal formula is:

$$\frac{D \text{ (desired)}}{H \text{ (on hand)}} \times V \text{ (volume)} = \text{units/hour} (\# \text{ mL} \times \text{units/mL} = \text{dose})$$

Example:

Heparin 20,000 units in 500 mL D$_5$W is ordered to run at 1,000 units/hour. How will the I.V. pump be set?

$$\frac{20,000 \text{ units}}{500 \text{ mL}} = 40 \text{ units/mL}$$

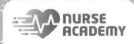

$$\frac{1,000 \text{ units (D)}}{40 \text{ units (H)}} \times 1 \text{ mL (V)} = X$$

Answer: X = 25 mL/hour

Example:

Heparin 20,000 units in 500 mL D$_5$W is infusing at 20 mL/hour. At how many units/hour is the heparin infusing?

$$\frac{20,000 \text{ units}}{500 \text{ mL}} = 40 \text{ units/mL}$$

$$\frac{40 \text{ units}}{1 \text{ mL}} \longrightarrow \frac{20 \text{ mL}}{1 \text{ hour}} = X$$

Answer: X = 800 units/hour

Patient safety depends on accurate I.V. drug dosing; precise calculations are essential to this process. Nurses shouldn't be apprehensive when I.V. drug dosages are presented in practice. Use the simple calculations conveyed in this article as a first step.

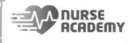

DOSAGE CALCULATIONS

I n this chapter, we will look at drug calculations. It's important to note that any time we do calculations we must have our measures in the same system and units. We will use the metric system as our common system.

Below are a few conversions related to the metric system, the basic units are the meter (m), liter (L), and gram (g, gm, or Gm).

Standard Units:

1 milligram (mg) = 1000 micrograms (mcg) or 0.001 grams (g)

1 g = 1000 mg

1 kilogram (kg) = 1000 g

1 kg = 2.2 pound (lb)

1 liter (L) = 1000 milliliters (mL)

If in your calculations you are required to convert larger values and units to smaller ones, multiply by 1000, or move the decimal point three places to the right,

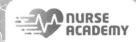

while to change to larger units, divide by 1000, or move the decimal point three places to the left.

FORMULAS FOR CALCULATING MEDICATION DOSAGE

BASIC FORMULA

$$\frac{D}{A} \times Q = X$$

Where D indicates the desired dosage ordered by the physician and A, the available dosage strength stated on the medication label. Q (quantity) is the volume in which the dosage strength is available (e.g., tablets, capsules, milliliters).

Example:

Ceclor 0.5 g PO b.i.d is the available order and 250 mg capsules. The first step is to get the same units of measurement. We already have 250 mg capsules; we need to change the ordered dose to mg. Therefore, we move the decimal point three places to the right, so the dosage to give is 500 mg.

$$\frac{D}{A} \times Q = X \qquad \frac{500 \text{ mg}}{250 \text{ mg}} \times 1 \text{ capsule} = 2 \text{ capsules}$$

When the left side represents known quantities, the dose on hand (H), and the vehicle (V), such as tablets, capsules, milliliters; and the right side represents the

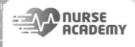

desired dose (D) and (X) the unknown amount to be given, we multiply the means (V and D), and the extremes (H and X), then solve for X.

Where we need to give Ceclor 0.5 g PO b.i.d., and we have 250 mg capsules available, we do the following:

First, convert to similar measures.

$$\frac{H}{V} = \frac{D}{X}$$

$$\frac{250 \text{ mg}}{1 \text{ capsule}} = \frac{500 \text{ mg}}{X \text{ capsules}}$$

1 capsule × 500 mg = 250 mg × X

500 = 250X

2 = X

Therefore, we will administer 2 capsules for our dose

FORMULAS FOR IV INFUSION

Flow Rate

$$\frac{\text{Total Volume in mL} \times \text{Drop Factor}}{\text{Time in minutes}} = \text{Drops per minute}$$

This formula can be used whenever we use a gravity infusion. Remember the time should always be in minutes and the volume always in mL.

To give 1000 mL of D5W over 24 hours, the tubing has a drop factor of 20 gtt/mL. The total volume is in Ml and we won't have to change that, but the time is in hours.

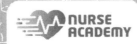

To convert our time to minutes, multiply it by 60. The total time in minutes will be 1440.

$$\frac{1000 \text{ mL} \times 20 \text{ gtt/mL}}{1440 \text{ minutes}} = \text{Drops per minute}$$

$$\frac{20,000}{1440} = 13.89, \text{ so we will run our infusion at 14 gtt/min}$$

When giving 3 L of NS over 24 hours, the tubing has a drop factor of 15 gtt/ml. Change the 3 L to mL by moving the decimal point (3000 mL) and time to minutes (24 hours = 1440 minutes).

$$\frac{3000 \text{ mL} \times 15 \text{ gtt/mL}}{1440 \text{ minutes}} = \frac{45,000}{1440} = 31.25 \text{ gtt/min} = 31 \text{ gtt/min for our rate.}$$

Flow Rate for Infusion Pumps

$$\frac{\text{Volume to be infused in mL}}{\text{Time in hours}} = \text{mL per hour}$$

For most infusion pumps it is necessary to program mL per hour. This formula makes it easier to calculate.

Give 1000 mL of D5W over 24 hours.

$$\frac{1000 \text{ mL}}{24 \text{ hours}} = \text{mL/hr} = 41.6 \text{ ml/hr} = 42 \text{ ml/hr for our pump rate}$$

Give 3L of NS over 24 hours. Change to mL (3000).

$$\frac{3000 \text{ mL}}{24 \text{ hours}} = 125 \text{ mL/hr}$$

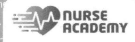

COMPLEX CALCULATIONS

For IV therapy there are more complex calculations that have to be done. These are referred to as titrations. You can use some of the basic formulas to achieve this but also involve multiple steps that must be followed depending on what has to be administered.

Calculating Units per Hour (U/h)

200 units of regular insulin is added to 500 mL of .9% NS. The order states infusing the regular insulin IV at 10 U/h. How many mL/h should the IV pump be set at?

The first step is to identify how many units of insulin are in each mL.

$$\frac{250\ U}{500\ mL} = \frac{X\ units}{1\ mL}$$

$500X = 200$

$X = 0.4$ units/mL

Run the drip at 10 U per hour, how many mL will contain 10 U?

$$\frac{1\ mL}{0.4\ U} = \frac{X\ mL}{10\ U}$$

$0.4\ X = 10$

$X = 25$ mL

There are 10 U of insulin in every 25 mL of fluid, run the pump at 25 mL per hour.

Another example:

20,000 units of heparin have been added to 500 mL of D5W. The order is to infuse

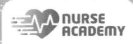

the heparin drip at 2000 U/h. How many mL/h will we set our pump for?

Step one, find out how many units of heparin are in each mL.

$$\frac{20{,}000\ U}{500\ mL} = \frac{X\ U}{1\ mL}$$

500X = 20,000

X = 40 units/mL

How many mL contain the ordered 2000 U?

$$\frac{1\ mL}{40\ U} = \frac{X\ mL}{2000\ U}$$

40 X = 2000

X = 50 mL

Run the pump at 50 mL/h.

Calculating by Microgram per Kilogram per Minute (mcg/kg/min)

$$\frac{\text{Ordered mcg/kg/min} \times \text{Patient weight in kg} \times 60\ \text{minutes/h}}{\text{Medication concentration (mcg/1 mL)}} = \text{mL/h}$$

Add 800 mg of dopamine to 250 ml of .9% Ns. Begin the infusion at 3 mcg/kg/minute. The patient's weight is 70 kg. Find the mL/hour to set the IV pump at.

Begin by identifying the concentration of the solution. There is 800 mg in 250 mL. Remember you need like units. Change the mg to mcg by moving the decimal point three places to the right.

The solution, therefore, has 800,000 mcg in 250 mL.

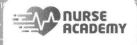

$$\frac{800,000 \text{ mcg}}{250 \text{ mL}} = \frac{X \text{ mcg}}{1 \text{ mL}}$$

250X = 800,000

X= 3200 mcg/mL

(Keep the number)

The order is for 3 mcg/kg/min. The patient weighs 70 kg. Multiply 70 by 3 to find the total mcg/min. 70 × 3 = 210, this results to 210 mcg/min.

The pump rate is always mL/hour, multiply the mcg/min by 60 to get mcg/h.

210 × 60 = 12,600, you will give 12,600 mcg/h.

Find out how many mL contain our 12,600 mcg. Use the concentration number that was saved earlier.

$$\frac{12,600 \text{ mcg}}{X \text{ mL}} = \frac{3200 \text{ mcg}}{1 \text{ mL}}$$

3200 X = 12,600

X = 3.9 mL

The IV pump rate will be 4 mL/hour.

Another example:

Propofol is ordered at 30 mcg/kg/min. The propofol concentration is 15 mg/mL. The patient weighs 75 kg. How many mL/h should the IV pump be programmed at?

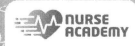

First, convert the units to be the same. If there is 15 mg/mL, that means there is 15,000 mcg/mL.

The order is for 30 mcg/kg/min.

The weight is 75 kg, so 75 × 30 = 2,250, this will give 2,250 mcg/min.

Pumps are always mL/h, so:

2250 mcg/min × 60 minutes/h = 135,000 mcg/h.

There is 15,000 mcg/mL, and need 135,000 mcg/hour, to find the mL/h:

$$\frac{1\ mL}{15,000\ mcg} = \frac{X\ mL}{135,000\ mcg}$$

15,000 X = 135,000

X = 9

The pump rate will be 9 Ml/hr.

Calculating Microgram per Minute (mcg/min)

$$\frac{Ordered\ mcg/min \times 60\ min/h}{Medication\ concentration\ (mcg/mL)} = mL/h$$

50 mg of nitroglycerin is added to 500 mL of .9% NS. The order is to infuse the nitroglycerin at 5 mcg/min. Calculate how many mL/h the IV pump needs to be set at.

First, calculate the mcg of the solution. If there is 50 mg in 500 mL, by moving the decimal point three spots to the right we will have 50,000 mcg in 500 mL.

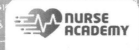

To calculate concentration:

$$\frac{50,0000 \text{ mcg}}{500\text{mL}} = \frac{X \text{ mgc}}{1 \text{ mL}}$$

500 X = 50,000

so X = 100 mcg/mL

$$\frac{5 \text{ mcg/min} \times 60 \text{ min/h}}{100 \text{ mcg/mL}} = X \text{ ml/h} \qquad \frac{300}{100} = X$$

X = 3 mL/h

Calculating milligrams per minute (mg/min)

$$\frac{\text{Desired mg/min} \times 60 \text{ min/h}}{\text{Medication concentration (mcg/mL)}} = \text{mL/h}$$

Lidocaine 1 g is added to 500 mL of D5W. The order desires to infuse the lidocaine at 2 mg/min. Calculate the mL/h for the infusion pump.

First, find the like units – 1 g in 500 mL = 1000 mg in 500 ml.

Calculate the concentration:

$$\frac{100 \text{ mg}}{500 \text{ mL}} = \frac{X \text{ mg}}{1 \text{ mL}}$$

500 X = 1000

X = 2 mg/mL

$$\frac{2 \text{ mg/min} \times 60 \text{ min/h}}{2 \text{ mg/ml}} = \frac{120}{2} = 60 \text{ mL/h}$$

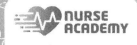

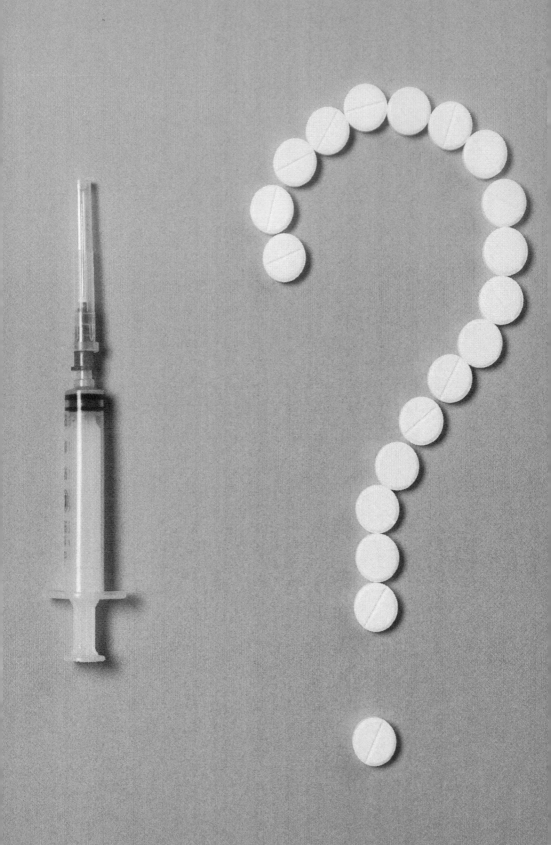

FLOW RATE CALCULATION

DEFINING FLOW RATE

Most calculations in nursing include finding volumes needed for oral or injected doses as well as working out IV infusion flow and drip rates. These calculations require the application of the various math skills looked at before. In this chapter, you will learn how to calculate the flow rate of IV infusions in mL/h, calculate IV infusion drip rates, and find the volume and time of IV infusions.

In physics, 'flow rate' would be defined as the rate through which a volume of fluid flows through a closed container and measured in GPM (gallon per minute) a unit of volumetric flow rate.

However, when applied to health and nursing, 'flow rate' would be defined as the number of heartbeats per unit of time, usually expressed or written as number per minute. A normal resting heart rate for an adult is 60-100 beats per minute.

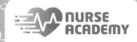

Most types of medications are delivered as continuous IV infusions in acute, ambulatory, long-term, home care, and critical care settings.

For a continuous IV medication, the type of administration system relies on factors like age and acuity of the patient, the type of medication ordered, the organization's practice, and the setting.

Flow rate devices range from simple mechanical devices using gravity to computerized smart electronic infusion devices. Without considering the type of administration system used to administer the continuous IV infusion, the goal is to control the rate of flow. Whether the medication is simple or complex, it must be taken and seen as an enhancement of patient care.

A continuous IV infusion is an infusion of medication in a solution into the venous system that is often used when the medication needs to be greatly diluted, the drug level in the blood must be tightly controlled, or large volumes of fluids need to be infused.

COMPONENTS OF DRUG CALCULATIONS

The universally accepted system of measurement for calculating drug dosages is the metric system. These measurements include:

- The amount of drug to be given (G) or desired dose: the amount of medication to be administered over a certain length of time.

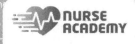

- Dose ordered (D): the amount of medication prescribed (e.g., 2.5 mg)

- Strength on hand (H): the medication available (e.g., 400 mg)

- Volume on hand (V): the amount of solution available for dilution (e.g., 400 mg/2 ml indicates 400 mg of medication in 2 ml of liquid volume)

- The concentration of a drug (C): the amount of medication diluted in a volume of IV solution (e.g., 400 mg dopamine/250 ml)

- Flow rate: the speed at which the IV fluid infuses expressed as volume over time (e.g., 20 ml/hr.)

- Drop factor: the number of drops in the IV drip chamber that is equivalent to 1 ml

- Length of administration

- Conversion factors

As discussed in the previous chapters, all units of measure used in the formula must be the same when calculations are performed. If they are not, the units of measure have to be converted.

POUNDS TO KILOGRAMS

Medication dosages based on weight are calculated using kilograms and not pounds.

The universal conversion formula is:

1 kg = 2.2 lb.

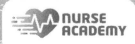

CALCULATING THE FLOW RATE

Below are ways to calculate flow rate and drop rate:

FLOW RATE

For electronic infusion controllers, the flow rate has to be set.

The rate is the volume in ml divided by the duration in hours (mls per hour).

Flow rate = Volume (ml) / Time (hours)

DROP RATE

For manual infusion controllers, the drop rate is set per minute (drops per minute).

Drop rate = Drop factor x Volume/60 x Time (hours)

In some controllers, the size of each drop of liquid is controlled by the internal mechanics which are usually fixed and cannot be altered.

This constant quality gives rise to the drop factor:

Drop factor = the number of drops it takes to make up one ml of fluid.

Two common sizes are:

- 20 drops per ml (typically for clear fluids)
- 15 drops per ml (typically for thicker substances, such as blood)

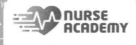

CALCULATING THE DURATION

OF AN INFUSION

A physician may have to calculate the duration an infusion will last.

Example:

How long will a 100ml infusion of sodium bicarbonate last if it is running at 42 drops per minute?

Let's assume the drop factor for the equipment is 20 drops per ml.

First, find out how many milliliters are transfused per minute:

- The drop rate is 42 drops per minute
- The drop factor is 20 drops per ml
- If we divide 42 drops per minute by 20 drops per milliliter, we'll find out the number of milliliters per minute
- 42/20 = 2.1 ml per minute

Divide the overall infusion of 100ml by the milliliters transfused per minute to get the answer:

100 ml / 2.1 ml per minute = 47.6 minutes

Depending on the type of pump used and medication to be administered, a flow rate or a drip rate may need to be calculated to set up an infusion.

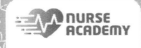

DETERMINING A DRUG DOSAGE

RATIO-PROPORTION METHOD:

H:V = D:G

$$\frac{\text{Drug on hand}}{\text{Volume of the drug on hand}} = \frac{\text{Dose ordered}}{\text{Amount to give}}$$

FORMULA METHOD:

$$\text{Amount to give (G)} = \frac{\text{Dose ordered (D)}}{\text{Strength on Hand (H)}} \times \text{Volume (V)}$$

There are several formulas that can be used to calculate drug dosages.

The following information is required for each:

- Amount of drug to be given (G)

- Dose ordered (D)

- Strength on hand (H)

- Volume on hand (V)

The above methods can be used here:

Example:

A vial contains clindamycin 600 mg/4 ml and the order is for 300 mg of clindamy-cin, Determine the Volume to be given.

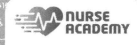

Ratio-Proportion Method

A ratio compares two related items while the proportion is the equality of two ratios.

H (mg): V (ml) = D (mg):G (ml)

600 mg:4 ml = 300 mg:G

(4 ml × 300 mg) equals the product of the extremes (600 mg × G):

1. Multiply the extremes (600 ~~mg~~ × G)

2. Multiply the means (4 ml × 300 ~~mg~~)

3. 600 G = 1200 ml

4. G = 1200 ÷ 600

5. G = 2 ml clindamycin

Total amount of drug (mg) ÷ total volume of solution (ml) = concentration of the solution (mg/ml)

DETERMINING DRUG CONCENTRATION

Concentration is the amount of medication per milliliter of fluid or by a fraction, a percentage of solution, or mass.

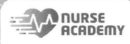

MG/ML

1. Determine the concentration of the drug.

    Total mg of drug ÷ total volume of solution (ml) = concentration of the solution (mg/ml)

2. Determine the infusion rate.

    Desired amount of drug (mg/min) ÷ concentration of solution (mg/ml) = infusion rate (ml/min)

3. Convert to ml/hr: ml/min × 60 min/hr = ml/hr

PERCENTAGE BY MASS

A percentage solution is a measure based on parts of 100. The conversion factor is 1% solution = 1 gm of the drug in 100 ml of solution.

$$\frac{\text{Mass of medication}}{\text{The mass of fluid}} \times 100$$

To determine the percentage by mass of a 100-gm sodium chloride solution containing 20 gm of medication, the nurse would apply the formula as follows:

20 gm of medication/100 gm of solution × 100

20%

PERCENTAGE BY VOLUME

$$\frac{\text{Volume of medication}}{\text{Total volume of solution}} \times 100\%$$

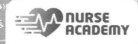

A 1000-ml bag of fluid contains 50 ml of medication. To determine the percentage by volume, the nurse would apply the formula as follows:

$$\frac{50 \text{ ml (volume of medication)}}{1000 \text{ ml (total volume of solution)}} \times 100\%$$

$(50 \div 1000) \times 100\% = 5\%$

TIME OF ADMINISTRATION

$$\frac{\text{Volume to be infused (ml)}}{\text{milliliters/hour (ml/hr)}} = \text{number of hours for infusion}$$

An infusion of D5W in 0.45% sodium chloride solution has 600 ml remaining in the medication container.

The rate of flow is 20 drops/min, and the drop factor is 12 drops/ml.

To determine how many hours it will take for the medication to infuse, the nurse follows these steps:

Convert 600 ml to hours.

$$\frac{600 \text{ ml} \times x \text{ drops} \times x \text{ min} \times x \text{ hours}}{x \text{ ml} \times x \text{ drops} \times x \text{ min}}$$

$$\frac{600 \text{ ml} \times 12 \text{ drops} \times 1 \text{ min} \times 1 \text{ hr}}{1 \text{ ml} \times 20 \text{ drops} \times 60 \text{ min}} = \frac{7200 \text{ hr}}{1200} = 6 \text{ hr}$$

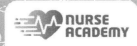

FLOW RATE CONVERSION CALCULATIONS

ML/MIN TO DROPS/MIN

A patient is to receive 240 ml of medication over 30 minutes. The drop factor of the IV administration set is 20 drops/ml. The nurse would determine the drops/min as follows:

$$\frac{240 \text{ ml}}{30 \text{ min}} \times \frac{20 \text{ drops}}{1 \text{ ml}} = \frac{4800 \text{ drops}}{30 \text{ min}} = 160 \text{ drops min(mU)/min to micro drops/min}$$

A patient is to receive 1000 ml of D5W with 10 units of oxytocin at 10 mU/min. The drop factor of the IV administration set tubing is 60 microdrops/ml. The nurse would determine the microdrops/min as follows:

1. Identify the conversion factor: 1000 mU = 1 unit (u)

2. Change the rate of flow from mU/min to microdrops/min:

$$\frac{10 \text{ mU}}{1 \text{ min}} \times \frac{x \text{ U}}{x \text{ mU}} \times \frac{x \text{ mL}}{x \text{ U}} \times \frac{x \text{ microdrops}}{x \text{ mL}} = \frac{\text{microdrops}}{\text{min}}$$

3. Identify known information:

   1000 mU = 1 u, 1000 ml = 10 u, and 60 micro drops = 1 ml.

4. Set up the equation with known information:

$$\frac{10 \text{ mU}}{1 \text{ min}} \times \frac{1 \text{ U}}{1000 \text{ mU}} \times \frac{1000 \text{ mL}}{10 \text{ U}} \times \frac{60 \text{ microdrops}}{1 \text{ mL}}$$

5. 60 microdrops/min

   D5W, 5% dextrose in water; mU, milliunits.

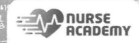

METRIC CONVERSIONS

WEIGHT

1 kilogram	× 1000	=	1000 grams
1 gram	× 1000	=	1000 milligrams
1 milligram	× 1000	=	1000 micrograms
1 microgram	÷ 1000	=	0.001 milligram
1 milligram	÷ 1000	=	0.001 gram
1 gram	÷ 1000	=	0.001 kilogram

VOLUME

1 liter	× 1000	=	1000 milliliters
1 milliliter	÷ 1000	=	0.001 liter

METRIC SYSTEM ABBREVIATIONS

WEIGHT	VOLUME	LENGTH
Kilogram = kg	Liter = L	Centimeter = cm
Gram = gm	Milliliter = ml	Millimeter = mm
Milligram = mg	Cubic centimeter = cc	
Microgram = mc		

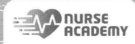

DETERMINING FLOW RATE

The units of measure for the flow rate may be ml/hr, ml/min, or drops/min.

FLOW RATE/HOUR:

Total volume (ml) ÷ administration time (hr) = milliliters/hour (ml/hr)

FLOW RATE/MINUTE:

Milliliters/hour (ml/hr) ÷ minutes/hour (min/hr) (60) = milliliters/minute (ml/min)

DROPS/MINUTE:

Milliliters/minute (ml/min) × drop factor = drops/minute (drops/min)

The three methods below can be used to answer this question: If the practitioner orders 2000 ml of medication to infuse over 24 hours, what is the flow rate?

FLOW RATE DETERMINATION

FLOW RATE/HR

Total volume (ml) ÷ administration time (hr) = ml/hr

2000 ml ÷ 24 hr = 83.3 ml/hr (round to nearest whole number for gravity administration)

Flow rate = 83 ml/hr

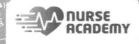

FLOW RATE/MIN

ml/hr ÷ 60 min per hr = ml/min

83 ml ÷ 60 min = 1.38 ml/min (round to nearest whole number for gravity administration)

Flow rate/min = 1 ml/min

DROPS/MIN

ml/min × drops/ml = drops/min

If the drop factor is 15 drops/ml:

$$\frac{1.4 \cancel{ml}}{min} \times \frac{15 \text{ drops}}{1 \cancel{ml}} = \frac{21 \text{ drops}}{min} = 21 \text{ drops/min}$$

HOURLY RATE DETERMINATION

(Drops/min × 60 min/hr) = ml/hr

DROP FACTOR

For an administration set with a drop factor of 15 drops/ml that is infusing a solution at a rate of 25 drops/min:

$$\frac{25 \text{ drops/min} \times 60 \text{ min/hr}}{15 \text{ drops/ml}} = \frac{ml}{hr}$$

$$\frac{1500}{15} = 100 \text{ ml/hr}$$

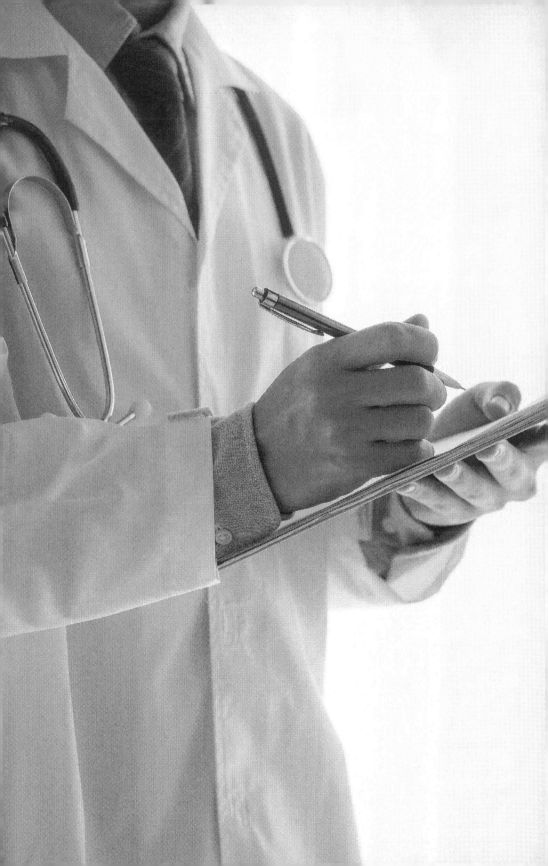

PERCENT AND RATIO STRENGTH CALCULATION

R atio strength is a ratio in the form of 1 in r. The corresponding fraction would have a numerator of 1. The current agreed convention is that when a ratio strength represents a solid in a liquid, we use grams for the solid and milliliters for the liquid.

Most prescriptions received at the Pharmacy have amounts of active ingredients expressed in percentage form, unlike weights and volumes which can be measured. Physicians know each active ingredient administered in certain percentage strengths will give the desired therapeutic effect.

Instead of calculating the amount of each needed ingredient for the prescription, a physician will indicate the percentage strength desired for each ingredient and expect the pharmacy to calculate the amount of each ingredient based on its percentage strength.

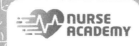

The percentage values on a prescription must be changed to amounts that can be weighed or measured. For the purposes of computation, percentages are usually changed to equivalent decimal fractions and are made by dropping the percent sign (%) and dividing the expressed numerator by 100.

CHANGING A DECIMAL TO A PERCENTAGE

The decimal is multiplied by 100 and the percent sign is affixed as a convenient means of expressing the concentration of active or inactive material in a pharmaceutical preparation.

PERCENTAGE WEIGHT-IN-VOLUME

In a true expression of percentage (i.e., parts per one hundred parts), the percentage of a liquid preparation (e.g., solution, suspension, lotion, etc.) would represent the grams of solute or constituent in 100 g of the liquid preparation. A different definition of percentage for solutions and other liquid preparations: represent grams of a solute or constituent in 100 mL of solution or liquid preparation.

The "correct" strength of a 1% (w/v) solution or other liquid preparation is defined as containing 1 g of the constituent in 100 mL of product. This variance to the definition of true percentage is based on an assumption that the solution/liquid preparation has a specific gravity of 1, as if it were water.

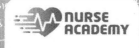

Each 100 mL of solution/liquid preparation is presumed to weigh 100 g and thus is used as the basis for calculating percentage weight-in-volume (e.g., 1% w/v = 1% of [100 mL taken to be] 100 g = 1 g in 100 mL).

WEIGHT OF ACTIVE INGREDIENT IN A SPECIFIC VOLUME, GIVEN ITS PERCENTAGE WEIGHT-IN-VOLUME

Taking water to represent any solvent or vehicle, we may prepare weight-in-volume percentage solutions or liquid preparations by the metric system if we use the following rule:

Multiply the required number of milliliters by the percentage strength, expressed as a decimal, to obtain the number of grams of solute or constituent in the solution or liquid preparation.

Volume (mL) X % (expressed as a decimal) = g of solute or constituent

Example:

How many grams of dextrose are required to prepare 4000 mL of a 5% solution?

4000 mL represent 4000 g of solution

5% = 0.05

0.05 = 200 g

Or, solving by dimensional analysis:

5 g/100 mL × 4000 mL = 200 g, answer.

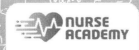

Examples:

How many grams of potassium permanganate should be used in compounding the following prescription?

Potassium Permanganate 0.02%

Purified Water ad   250.0 mL

Sig. As directed.

250 mL represent 250 g of solution

0.02% = 0.0002

X 0.0002 = 0.05 g, answer.

How many grams of aminobenzoic acid should be used in preparing 8 fluid ounces of a 5% solution in 70% alcohol?

8 fl. oz. = 8 × 29.57 mL = 236.56 mL

236.56 mL represents 236.56 g of solution

5 %= 0.05

X 0.05 = 11.83 g, answer.

PERCENTAGE WEIGHT-IN-VOLUME OF SOLUTION, GIVEN WEIGHT OF SOLUTE OR CONSTITUENT AND VOLUME OF SOLUTION OR LIQUID PREPARATION

Example:

What is the percentage strength (w/v) of a solution of urea, if 80 mL contains 12g?

80 mL of water weigh 80 g

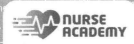

X = (12 g/80g) × 100%

X=15%, answer.

VOLUME OF SOLUTION OR LIQUID PREPARATION, GIVEN PERCENTAGE STRENGTH WEIGHT-IN-VOLUME AND WEIGHT OF SOLUTE

Example:

How many milliliters of a 3% solution can be made from 27 g of ephedrine sulfate?

X g / 27 g = 3%

x = 900 g, weight of the solution if it were water Volume (in mL) = 900 mL

Liquids are usually measured by volume; the percentage strength indicates the number of parts by volume of the active ingredient contained in the total volume of the solution or liquid preparation considered as 100 parts by volume.

If there is any possibility of misinterpretation, this kind of percentage should be specified: e.g., 10 %(v/v).

VOLUME OF ACTIVE INGREDIENT IN A SPECIFIC VOLUME, GIVEN PERCENTAGE STRENGTH VOLUME-IN-VOLUME

Example:

How many milliliters of liquefied phenol should be used in compounding the following prescription?

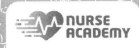

Liquefied Phenol   2.5%

Calamine Lotion ad   240.0 mL

Sig. For external use.

Volume (mL) × % (expressed as a decimal) = milliliters of active ingredient

240 mL × 0.025= 6 mL

Or, solving by dimensional analysis:

(2.5 mL / 100 mL) × 240 mL = 6 mL

PERCENTAGE VOLUME-IN-VOLUME OF SOLUTION OR LIQUID PREPARATION, GIVEN VOLUME OF ACTIVE INGREDIENT AND VOLUME OF SOLUTION

The required volumes may be calculated from given weights and specific gravities.

Example:

In preparing 250 mL of a certain lotion, a pharmacist used 4 mL of liquefied phenol. What was the percentage (v/v) of liquefied phenol in the lotion?

X = (4 mL / 250 mL) × 100%

X = 1.6%, answer.

What is the percentage strength (v/v) of a solution of 800 g of a liquid with a specific gravity of 0.800 in enough water to make 4000 mL?

800 g of water measure 800 mL

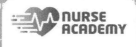

800 g ÷ 0.800 = 1000 mL of active ingredient

X = (1000 mL / 4000 mL) × 100%

X = 25%, answer.

Or, solving by dimensional analysis:

$$\frac{800 \text{ mL}}{0.800} \times \frac{1}{4000 \text{ mL}} \times 100\% = 25\%, \text{ answer}$$

This may require first determining the volume of the active ingredient from its weight and specific gravity.

Examples:

Peppermint spirit contains 10% (v/v) of peppermint oil. What volume of the spirit will contain 75 mL of peppermint oil?

10% = 75 mL / X mL

X = 750 mL, answer.

TRUE PERCENTAGE OR PERCENTAGE BY WEIGHT

This indicates the number of parts by weight of active ingredient contained in the total weight of the solution or mixture considered as 100 parts by weight.

Liquids are not customarily measured by weight. Therefore, a weight-in-weight solution or liquid preparation of a solid or a liquid in a liquid should be so designated: e.g., 70% (w/w).

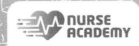

Weight of Active Ingredient in a Specific Weight of Solution or Liquid Preparation, Given its Weight-in-Weight Percentage Strength.

How many grams of phenol should be used to prepare 240 g of a 0.5% (w/w) solution in water?

Weight of solution (g) × % (expressed as a decimal) = g of solute

240 g × 0.05 = 12 g

CALCULATING PERCENTAGE STRENGTH WEIGHT-IN-WEIGHT

If the weight of the finished solution or liquid preparation is not given when calculating its percentage strength, other data must be supplied from which it may be calculated:

- the weights of both ingredients
- the volume and the specific gravity of the solution or liquid preparation

Examples:

If 1,500 g of a solution contains 75 g of a drug substance, what is the percentage strength (wlw) of the solution?

$$\frac{1500 \text{ g}}{75 \text{ g}} = \frac{100 \text{ %}}{\text{X %}}$$

X = 5%, answer

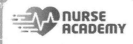

If 5 g of boric acid is added to 100 mL of water, what is the percentage strength (w/w) of the solution?

100 mL of water weigh 100 g

100 g + 5 g = 105 g, weight of solution

$$X = \frac{5\ g}{105\ g} \times 100\%$$

X = 4.76%, answer.

RATIO STRENGTH

The concentration of weak solutions or liquid preparations is frequently expressed in terms of ratio strength. Ratio strength is merely another way of expressing the percentage strength of solutions or liquid preparations (and, less frequently, of mixtures of solids).

For example,

5% means 5 parts per 100 or 5:100

Although 5 parts per 100 designates a ratio strength, it is customary to translate this designation into a ratio; thus, 5:100 = 1: 20.

1/1000, used to designate a concentration, is to be interpreted as:

- For solids in liquids = 1 g of solute or constituent in 1000 mL of solution or liquid preparation.

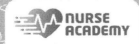

- For liquids in liquids = 1 mL of constituent in 1000 mL of solution or liquid preparation.
- For solids in solids = 1 g of constituent in 1000 g of mixture.

The ratio and percentage strengths of any solution or mixture of solids are proportional, and either is easily converted to the other by the use of proportion.

RATIO STRENGTH GIVEN AS PERCENTAGE STRENGTH

Express 0.02% as a ratio strength.

$$\frac{0.2\%}{100\%} = \frac{1 \text{ part}}{X \text{ parts}}$$

X = 5000

Ratio strength = 1 : 5000, answer.

PERCENTAGE STRENGTH GIVEN AS RATIO STRENGTH

Express 1: 4000 as a percentage strength.

$$\frac{100\%}{X\%} = \frac{4000 \text{ parts}}{1 \text{ part}}$$

X = 0.025%, answer.

PROBLEMS INVOLVING RATIO STRENGTH

Translate the problem into one based on percentage strength. Solve it according to the rules and methods discussed under percentage preparations.

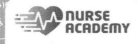

Examples:

How many grams of potassium permanganate should be used in preparing 500 mL of a 1:2500 solution?

1:2500 = 0.04%	Or,
500 (g) × 0.0004 = 0.2 g	1:2500 means 1 g in 2500 mL of solution
	$$\frac{2500\ mL}{500\ mL} = \frac{1\ g}{X\ g}$$
	X = 0.2, answer.

How many milligrams of gentian violet should be used in preparing the following solution?

Gentian Violet Solution   500 mL

1:10,000

Sig. Instill as directed.	Or,
1:10,000 = 0.01%	1:10,000 means
500 (g) × 0.0001 = 0.050 g or 50 mg	1 g of 10,000 mL of solution
	$$\frac{10,000\ mL}{500\ mL} = \frac{1\ g}{X\ g}$$
	X = 0.050 g, or 50 mg, answer.

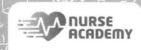

TYPES OF PERCENT

It is important to remember that percent means "parts per hundred" and is expressed in the following way:

OF PARTS 100 PARTS

Weight/Weight percent is the number of grams in 100 grams of a solid preparation.

Volume/Volume percent is defined as the number of milliliters in every 100 ml of solution.

When percentage type is not stated, this would mean that dilutions of:

- Dry ingredients in a dry preparation are percent W/W
- Dry ingredients in a liquid are percent W/V
- A liquid in a liquid is percent V/V

SOLVING PERCENTAGE PROBLEMS

ONE PERCENT METHOD:

The one percent method is used to calculate the amount of active ingredient when the final volume or weight of the preparation is known.

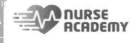

This method, however, cannot be used to calculate the amount of preparation that can be made when the percentage strength and the amount of active ingredient are known.

Formula:

(1 percent of the total amount of preparation) × (number of percent) = The amount of active ingredient)

DILUTION OF STOCK PREPARATIONS

Often, pharmacists will go to a stock solution to obtain the amount of active ingredient needed to make a preparation. This may happen if the amount required is too small to accurately weigh on a torsion balance.

It is easier to measure the amount of stock solution than set up a balance, weigh the ingredients, and compound the entire product. Stock preparations are an important aspect of pharmacy.

FORMULAS:

For these formulas to work:

- Volumes and weights must be expressed in the same units
- Concentrations must be expressed in the same units

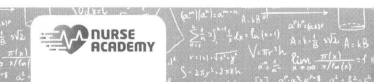

Formula:

$$V\,C = V_1\,C_1$$

Where:

V = Volume of stock preparation

C = Concentration of stock preparation

V_1 = Volume of desired preparation

C_1 = Concentration of desired preparation

Formula:

$$W\,C = W_1\,C_1$$

Where:

W = Weight of stock preparation

C = Concentration of stock preparation

W_1 = Weight of desired preparation

C_1 = Concentration of desired preparation

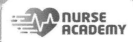

ALLIGATION

This is a method used in solving problems involved with mixing two products of different strengths to form a product having a desired intermediate strength.

It is used to calculate:

- The amount of diluent that has to be added to a given amount of higher strength preparation to make a desired lower strength.
- The amounts of active ingredient that must be added to a given amount of lower strength preparation to make a higher strength.
- The amount of higher and lower strength preparations that have to be combined to make the desired amount of an intermediate strength.

Often it is more practical to dilute known strength preparation than to compound the whole preparation. This may involve weighing, measuring, heating, levitating, and mixing of all the ingredients to achieve the finished product.

Sometimes, a simple calculation allows us to calculate the amount of diluent to be added to an already prepared higher strength preparation to form the strength desired. This would then be simplified by combining the two ingredients. Periodically, it is vital to increase the strength of a preparation by adding an active ingredient.

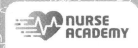

If a doctor is treating a patient with 1-percent coal tar ointment and he decides to increase the strength to 2 percent, it can be accomplished by adding an unknown amount of coal tar (100 percent). This would be due to the mixing of a higher and a lower strength to form an intermediate strength, the unknown amount may be found by using alligation.

FINDING PROPORTIONS

a. Draw a problem matrix

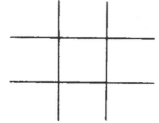

b. Insert quantities as shown

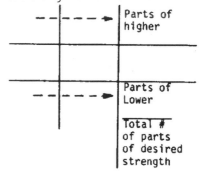

Higher strength

Desired strength

Lower strength

c. Subtract along the diagonals

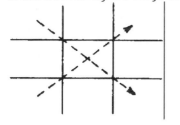

d. Read along the horizontals

Parts of higher

Parts of Lower

Total # of parts of desired strength

Remember that the desired strength goes in the center square of the matrix. This is the strength of the preparation that you want to make. Often, the strength of the prescription will be the desired strength.

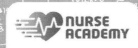

ALLIGATION PROBLEMS

Example 1: A pharmacist has a 70% alcoholic elixir and a 20% alcoholic elixir. He needs a 30% alcoholic elixir to use as a vehicle for medications. In what proportion must the 70% elixir and the 20% elixir be combined to make a 30% elixir?

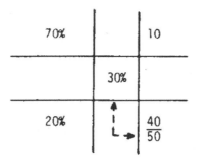

10 parts of 70%

Reduced:
1 part of 70 %

40 parts of 20%	4 parts of 20 %
50 parts of 30%	5 parts of 30 %

Note: This means that if one part of 70% elixir is mixed with four parts of 20% elixir, it will yield five parts of 30% elixir. The dotted arrows in the matrix above have been placed as a reminder that the total number of parts always represents the desired strength.

Example 2: In what proportion must plain coal tar be combined with a 2% coal tar ointment to make a 4% coal tar ointment?

Remember that coal tar, because it is pure coal tar and not diluted, will be a higher (100 percent) strength.

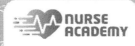

If one part of coal tar is combined with 48 parts of 2% coal tar ointment, it will yield 49 parts of 4% coal tar ointment.

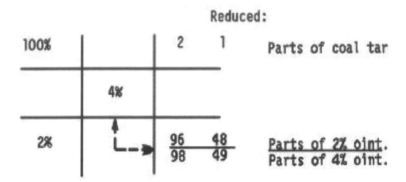

FORMULATING EQUATIONS USING MATRIX

Before the matrix is formed, the problem is analyzed to determine the method that is best for working the problem. The keywords which indicate that this is an alligation problem are 'must be added to'.

Other keywords indicating alligation as the best method include 'must be combined' and 'must be mixed'.

Example:

Determine the amount that must be added to 300 ml of 70% alcoholic solution to make a 40% alcoholic solution.

In this problem, 40% is the desired strength and must be placed in the center of the matrix. Seventy percent is a higher strength and must be placed in the upper

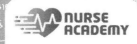

left-hand corner of the matrix. If no lower strength is given, it can be assumed to be 0%.

Reduced:

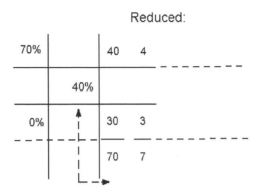

The relationship of the strength of the parts to their joined final volume may be used as the first ratio of a proportion.

Place the known factors in the proper position on the matrix. Assign the X value first to formulate the complete equation: The question seeks to determine the amount of water in millimeters; the X value is placed on the extended line oppo-site the percentage of alcohol denoted by water.

Reduced:

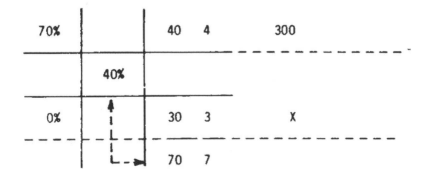

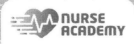

Another factor is that the water will be added to 300 ml of 70%. The 300-ml, because it pertains to the 70%, is placed on the line opposite the 70% on the matrix (see above). Once there are two values on the line and two values on another line, these values form the proportion.

IF

$$\frac{4}{3} = \frac{300}{X}$$

Cross Multiply:

4X = 900

X = 225 ml of 0% (Water)

Remember that, when distilled water, ointment bases, or normal saline are used as diluents, they will contain zero percent (0%) active ingredient.

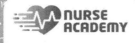

CONCLUSION

This course has offered ways and guidance that nursing students can apply in solving calculations. It has also provided evidence to emphasize the need for nurses to maintain competency during selected calculations. A variety of examples of calculation problems common in nursing practice have also been presented and solved.

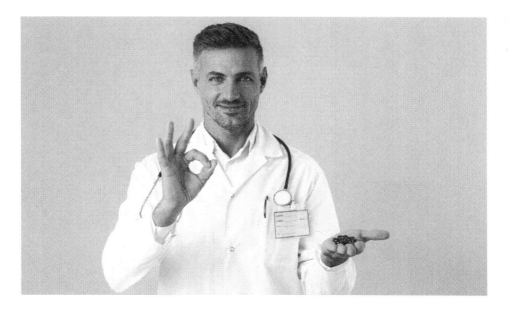

This course has provided the opportunity for practice with at least two methods for solving particular problems.

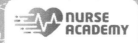

Made in the USA
Coppell, TX
05 October 2022

84135638R00061